Simple Keto Diet Cooking Guide Over 50

Quick and Tasty Keto Recipes for Women Over 50

Grace Studridge

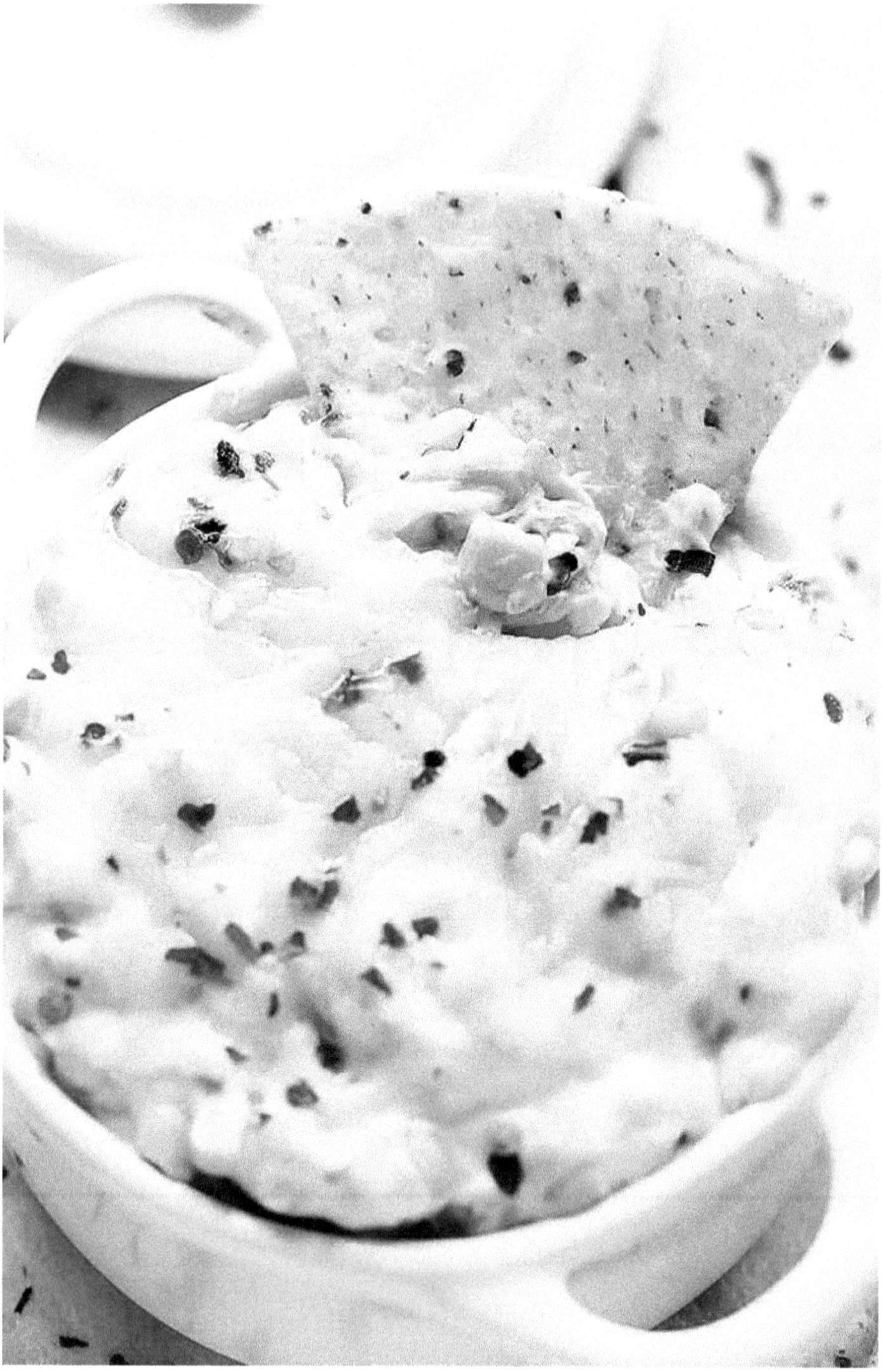

TABLE OF CONTENTS

Creamy Crab Dip

Preparation Time 5 minutes

Cooking Time: 10 minutes

Servings 12

Ingredients:

- Crab meat, chopped – 1 pound
- Chopped white onion – 2 tablespoons
- Minced garlic – 1 tablespoon
- Lemon juice – 2 tablespoons
- Cream cheese, cubed – 16 ounces
- Avocado mayonnaise – 1/3 cup
- Grape juice – 2 tablespoons

Directions:

1. Place all the ingredients for the dip in a medium bowl and stir until combined.
2. Divide dip evenly between small bowls and serve as a party dip.

Nutrition:

Calories: 100 | Fat: 4 | Fiber: 1 | Carbs: 4 | Protein: 4

Creamy Cheddar and Bacon Spread with Almonds

Preparation Time : 10 minutes

Cooking Time: 10 minutes

Servings 12

Ingredients:

- Bacon, cooked and chopped – 12 ounces
- Chopped sweet red pepper – 2 tablespoons
- Medium white onion, peeled and chopped – 1
- Salt – ¾ teaspoon
- Ground black pepper – ½ teaspoon
- Almonds, chopped – ½ cup
- Cheddar cheese, grated – 1 pound
- Avocado mayonnaise – 2 cups

Directions:

1. Place all the ingredients for the dip in a medium bowl and stir until combined.
2. Divide dip evenly between small bowls and serve as a party dip.

Nutrition:

calories: 184 | fat: 12 | fiber: 1 | carbs: 4 | protein: 5

Green Tabasco Devilled Eggs

Preparation Time : 20 minutes

Cooking Time: 10 minutes

Servings : 6

Ingredients:

- 6 Eggs
- 1/3 cup Mayonnaise
- 1 ½ tbsp. Green Tabasco
- Salt and Pepper, to taste

Directions:

1. Place the eggs in a saucepan over medium heat and pour boiling water over, enough to cover them.
2. Cook for 6-8 minutes.
3. Place in an ice bath to cool.
4. When safe to handle, peel the eggs and slice them in half.
5. Scoop out the yolks and place in a bowl.
6. Add the remaining ingredients.
7. Whisk to combine.
8. Fill the egg holes with the mixture.
9. Serve and enjoy!

Nutrition:

Calories 175 | Total Fats 17g | Net Carbs: 5g | Protein 6g | Fiber: 1g

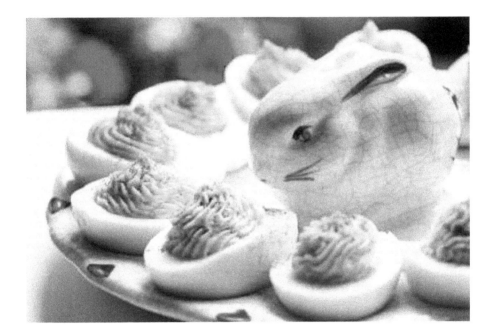

Herbed Cheese Balls

Preparation Time : 30 MIN

Cooking Time: 10 minutes

Servings : 20

Ingredients:

- 1/3 cup grated Parmesan Cheese
- 3 tbsp. Heavy Cream
- 4 tbsp. Butter, melted
- ¼ tsp Pepper
- 2 Eggs
- 1 cup Almond Flour
- ¼ cup Basil Leaves
- ¼ cup Parsley Leaves
- 2 tbsp. chopped Cilantro Leaves
- 1/3 cup crumbled Feta Cheese

Directions:

1. Place the ingredients in your food processor.
2. Pulse until the mixture becomes smooth.
3. Transfer to a bowl and freeze for 20 minutes or so, to set.
4. Shale the mixture into 20 balls.

5. Meanwhile, preheat the oven to 350 degrees F.

6. Arrange the cheese balls on a lined baking sheet.

7. Place in the oven and bake for 10 minutes.

8. Serve and enjoy!

Nutrition:

Calories 60 | Total Fats 5g | Net Carbs: 8g | Protein 2g | Fiber: 1g

Cheesy Salami Snack

Preparation Time : 30 MIN

Cooking Time: 10 minutes

Servings : 6

Ingredients:

- 4 ounces Cream Cheese
- 7 ounces dried Salami
- ¼ cup chopped Parsley

Directions:

1. Preheat the oven to 325 degrees F.
2. Slice the salami thinly (I got 30 slices).
3. Arrange the salami on a lined sheet and bake for 15 minutes.
4. Arrange on a serving platter and top each salami slice with a bit of cream cheese.
5. Serve and enjoy!

Nutrition:

Calories 139 | Total Fats 15g | Net Carbs: 1g | Protein 9g | Fiber: 0g

Pesto & Olive Fat Bombs

Preparation Time : 25 MIN

Cooking Time: 10 minutes

Servings : 8

Ingredients:

- 1 cup Cream Cheese
- 10 Olives, sliced
- 2 tbsp. Pesto Sauce
- ½ cup grated Parmesan Cheese

Directions:

1. Place all of the ingredients in a bowl.
2. Stir well to combine.
3. Place in the freezer and freeze for 15-20 minutes, to set.
4. Shape into 8 balls.
5. Serve and enjoy!

Nutrition:

Calories 123 | Total Fats 13g | Net Carbs: 3g | Protein 4g | Fiber: 3g

Cheesy Broccoli Nuggets

Preparation Time : 25 MIN

Cooking Time: 10 minutes

Servings : 4

Ingredients:

- 1 cup shredded Cheese
- ¼ cup Almond Flour
- 2 cups Broccoli Florets, steamed in the microwave for 5 minutes
- 2 Egg Whites
- Salt and Pepper, to taste

Directions:

1. Preheat the oven to 350 degrees F.
2. Place the broccoli florets in a bowl and mash them with a potato masher.
3. Add the remaining ingredients and mix well with your hands, until combined.
4. Line a baking sheet with parchment paper.
5. Drop 20 scoops of the mixture onto the sheet.
6. Place in the oven and bake for 20 minutes or until golden.

7. Serve and enjoy!

Nutrition:

Calories 145 | Total Fats 9g | Net Carbs: 4g | Protein 10g | Fiber: 1g

Salmon Fat Bombs

Preparation Time : 90 MIN

Cooking Time: 50 minutes

Servings : 6

Ingredients:

- ½ cup Cream Cheese
- 1 ½ tbsp. chopped Dill
- 1 ¾ ounces Smoked Salmon, sliced
- 1 tbsp. Lemon Juice
- 1/3 cup Butter
- ¼ tsp Red Pepper Flakes
- ¼ tsp Garlic Powder
- Pinch of Salt
- ¼ tsp Pepper

Directions:

1. Place the butter, salmon, lemon juice, and cream cheese, in your food processor.
2. Add the seasonings.
3. Pulse until smooth.
4. Drop spoonfuls of the mixture onto a lined dish.
5. Sprinkle with the dill.

6. Place in the fridge for about 80 minutes.

7. Serve and enjoy!

Nutrition:

Calories 145 | Total Fats 16g | Net Carbs: 7g | Protein 3g | Fiber: 1g

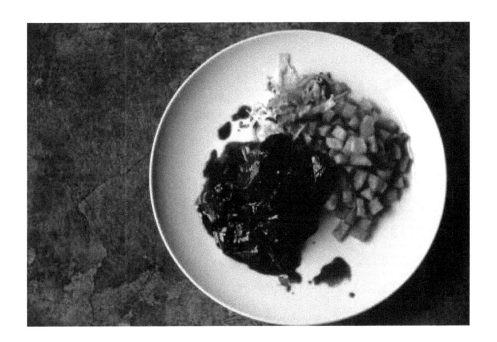

Guacamole Bacon Bombs

Preparation Time : 30 MIN

Cooking Time: 10 minutes

Servings : 6

Ingredients:

- 1 tsp minced Garlic
- ¼ cup Butter
- ½ Avocado, flesh scooped out
- 1 tbsp. Lime Juice
- 1 tbsp. chopped Cilantro
- 4 Bacon Slices, cooked and crumbled
- 3 tbsp. diced Shallots
- Salt and Pepper, to taste
- 1 tbsp. minced Jalapeno

Directions:

1. Place all of the ingredients, except the bacon, in your food processor.
2. Pulse until smooth. Alternatively, you can do this by whisking in a bowl. Just keep in mind that this way you will have chunks of garlic and jalapenos.
3. Transfer to a bowl and place in the freezer.

4. Freeze for 20 minutes, or until set.

5. Shape into 6 balls.

6. Coat them with bacon pieces.

7. Serve and enjoy!

Nutrition:

Calories 155 | Total Fats 15g | Net Carbs: 4g | Protein 4g | Fiber: 3g

Keto Cornbread

Preparation Time : 5 minutes;

Cooking Time : 2 minutes;

Servings : 2

Ingredients

- 1 ¾ oz almond flour
- ¼ tsp baking powder
- 1/8 tsp salt
- 1 tbsp. melted butter
- 1 egg

Directions:

1. Take a small bowl, place butter and egg in it, whisk until combined and then whisk in flour, baking powder, and salt until smooth batter comes together.
2. Take a small microwave proof container, spoon prepared batter in it, and then microwave for 1 minute and 45 seconds at high heat setting until cooked.
3. When done, cut bread into slices, then spread with butter and serve.

Nutrition :

116.2 Calories; 10.4 g Fats; 4.3 g Protein; 1.1 g Net Carb; 1.5 g Fiber;

Flax Seed Bread Sandwich

Preparation Time : 10 minutes;

Cooking Time : 10 minutes;

Servings : 2

Ingredients

- 4 oz ground flaxseed
- 2 tsp coconut flour
- ½ tsp baking soda
- 1 tsp apple cider vinegar
- 2 tbsp. almond milk, unsweetened
- Seasoning:
- ¼ tsp sesame seeds
- ¼ tsp pumpkin seeds
- ¼ tsp sunflower seeds
- Peanut butter for serving

Directions:

1. Take a medium bowl, place flaxseed in it, add flour, baking soda, vinegar, and milk and mix by using hand until smooth dough ball comes together.

2. Take a shallow dish, place sesame seeds, pumpkin seeds and sunflower seeds in it and then stir until mixed.
3. Divide dough ball into two pieces, roll each piece into a loaf and then press into seed mixture until evenly coated on both sides.
4. Place dough onto a heatproof plate, microwave for 1 minute and then cool breads for 5 minutes.
5. Slice each bread into half, then spread with peanut butter and serve.

Nutrition :

191 Calories; 15.1 g Fats; 4.8 g Protein; 1.2 g Net Carb; 7.1 g Fiber

Cheesy Jalapeno Cornbread

Preparation Time : 5 minutes;

Cooking Time : 2 minutes;

Servings : 2

Ingredients

- 1 jalapeno pepper, chopped
- 1 ¾ oz almond flour
- ¼ tsp baking powder
- 1 egg
- 1 tbsp. grated parmesan cheese
- Seasoning:
- 1 tbsp. melted butter
- 1/8 tsp salt
- 1/8 tsp ground black pepper

Directions:

1. Take a small bowl, place butter and egg in it, whisk until combined, and then whisk in remaining ingredients until smooth batter comes together.
2. Take a small microwave proof container, spoon prepared batter in it, and then microwave for 1

minute and 45 seconds at high heat setting until cooked.

3. When done, cut bread into slices, then spread with butter and serve.

Nutrition :

131 Calories; 11.1 g Fats; 4.8 g Protein; 1.1 g Net Carb; 0.9 g Fiber;

Cheese Cup

Preparation Time : 5 minutes;

Cooking Time : 5 minutes;

Servings : 2

Ingredients

- 4 tsp coconut flour
- 1/16 tsp baking soda
- 1 tbsp. grated mozzarella cheese
- 1 tbsp. grated parmesan cheese
- 2 eggs
- Seasoning:
- ¼ tsp salt
- ½ tsp dried basil
- ½ tsp dried parsley

Directions:

1. Take a medium bowl, place all the ingredients in it, and whisk until well combined.
2. Take two ramekins, grease them with oil, distribute the prepared batter in it and then microwave for 1 minute and 45 seconds until done.

3. When done, take out muffin from the ramekin, cut in half, and then serve.

Nutrition :

125 Calories; 8.1 g Fats; 9.5 g Protein; 1.1 g Net Carb; 1.7 g Fiber;

Cinnamon Mug Cake

Preparation Time : 5 minutes;

Cooking Time : 5 minutes;

Servings : 2

Ingredients

- 3 tbsp. almond flour
- 1 tbsp. erythritol sweetener
- 3 tbsp. butter, unsalted
- 2 tbsp. cream cheese
- 1 egg
- Seasoning:
- 1 tsp baking soda
- ¾ tsp cinnamon

Directions:

1. Take a heatproof mug, place 2 tbsp. butter in it, and then microwave for 30 seconds or more until butter melts.
2. Then add remaining ingredients, reserving cream cheese and remaining butter, stir until mixed and microwave for 1 minute and 20 seconds until done.

3. Run a knife along the side of the mug and then take out the cake.
4. Melt the remaining butter, top it over the cake, then top with cream cheese, cut cake in half, and serve.

Nutrition : 298 Calories; 28.8 g Fats; 6.7 g Protein; 1.3 g Net Carb; 1.7 g Fiber;

Spicy Dosa

Preparation Time : 5 minutes;

Cooking Time : 8 minutes;

Servings : 2

Ingredients

- oz almond flour
- ½ tsp ground cumin
- ½ tsp ground coriander
- oz grated mozzarella cheese
- 4 oz coconut milk, unsweetened
- Seasoning:
- ¼ tsp salt
- 2 tsp avocado oil

Directions:

1. Take a medium bowl, place all the ingredients in it except for oil, and stir until well combined and smooth batter comes together.

2. Take a medium skillet pan, place it over medium heat, add 1 tsp oil and when hot, pour in half of the prepared batter, spread it evenly in a circular shape,

then switch heat to the low level and cook for 2 minutes per side until golden brown and cooked.

3. Transfer dosa to a plate, then repeat with the remaining batter and serve.

Nutrition :

181 Calories; 16.5 g Fats; 6 g Protein; 2 g Net Carb; 0 g Fiber;

Garlic Cheese Balls

Preparation Time : 10 minutes;

Cooking Time : 0 minutes;

Servings : 2

Ingredients

- 2 bacon sliced, cooked, chopped
- ½ tsp minced garlic
- 2 oz cream cheese, softened
- 2 tbsp. sour cream
- 3 tbsp. grated parmesan cheese
- Seasoning:
- ½ tsp Italian seasoning

Directions:

1. Take a medium bowl, place cheese in it, then add remaining ingredients except for bacon and stir until mixed.
2. Cover the bowl, let it refrigerate for 1 hour until chilled, and then shape the mixture into four balls.
3. Roll the balls in chopped bacon until coated, refrigerate for 30 minutes until firm, and then serve.

Nutrition :

335 Calories; 28.7 g Fats; 12.4 g Protein; 5.8 g Net Carb; 0 g Fiber;

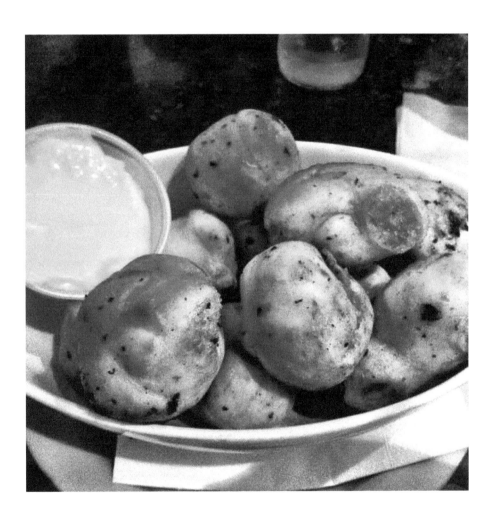

Cheddar and Green Onion Biscuits

Preparation Time : 5 minutes;

Cooking Time : 8 minutes;

Servings : 2

Ingredients

- 1 tsp chopped green onion
- 2 ½ tbsp. coconut flour
- 2 ½ tbsp. melted butter, unsalted
- 2 oz grated cheddar cheese
- 1 egg
- Seasoning:
- 1/8 tsp baking powder
- ½ tsp garlic powder
- ¼ tsp salt
- 1/8 tsp ground black pepper

Directions:

1. Turn on the oven, then set it to 400 degrees F and let it preheat.

2. Take a medium bowl, place flour in it, and then stir in garlic powder, baking powder, salt, and black pepper.
3. Take a separate medium bowl, crack the egg in it, whisk in butter until blended, and then whisk this mixture into the flour until incorporated and smooth.
4. Fold in green onion and cheese, then drop the mixture in the form of mounds onto a cookie sheet greased with oil and bake for 8 minutes until lightly browned.
5. When done, brush biscuit with some more melted butter and then serve.

Nutrition :

272 Calories; 23 g Fats; 11.5 g Protein; 4.5 g Net Carb; 0.7 g Fiber;

Basil Wrapped Cheese Balls

Preparation Time : 10 minutes;

Cooking Time : 0 minutes;

Servings : 2

Ingredients

- 2 oz grated cheddar cheese
- 3 oz grated mozzarella cheese
- 3 oz grated parmesan cheese
- ¼ tsp ground black pepper
- 8 basil leaves

Directions:

1. Take a medium bowl, place all the cheeses in it, add black pepper, stir until blended, then cover the bowl and let it refrigerate for 30 minutes until firm.

2. Then shape the mixture into 1-inch long eight balls, then place each ball on the wide end of a basil leaf and roll it up.

3. Serve immediately.

Nutrition :

428 Calories; 31.4 g Fats; 28.9 g Protein; 7.5 g Net Carb; 0 g Fiber;

Double Cheese Chips

Preparation Time : 10 minutes;

Cooking Time : 10 minutes;

Servings : 2

Ingredients

- 3 oz grated cheddar cheese
- 5 oz grated parmesan cheese
- 1/8 tsp onion powder
- 1/8 tsp ground cumin
- 1/8 tsp red chili powder
- Seasoning:
- 1/8 tsp salt

Directions:

1. Turn on the oven, then set it to 400 degrees F and let it preheat.
2. Take a medium bowl, place cheeses in it, add salt, onion powder, cumin, and red chili powder and stir until mixed.
3. Take a baking pan, line it with parchment paper, spread cheese mixture on it in an even layer, and then

bake for 10 minutes until cheese has melted and begin to crisp.

4. When done, remove the baking pan from the oven, let it cool completely and then cut it into triangles.

5. Serve.

Nutrition :

468 Calories; 34.2 g Fats; 30.3 g Protein; 9.3 g Net Carb; 0 g Fiber;

Bacon Caprese with Parmesan

Preparation Time : 5 minutes;

Cooking Time : 8 minutes;

Servings : 2

Ingredients

- 2 slices of bacon
- 2 Roma tomato, sliced
- 1 tsp balsamic vinegar
- 2 tbsp. avocado oil
- 1 tbsp. grated parmesan cheese
- Seasoning:
- ½ tsp salt
- ½ tsp ground black pepper

Directions:

1. Take a frying pan, place it over medium heat and when hot, add bacon and cook for 3 to 4 minutes until crispy.
2. Transfer bacon to a cutting board, let it cool for 5 minutes and then chop it.
3. Turn on the broiler and let it preheat.

4. Take a medium baking sheet, line it with aluminum foil, spray with oil, spread tomato slices on it, and then drizzle with vinegar and oil.

5. Season with salt and black pepper, sprinkle with cheese and bacon and then broil tomatoes for 1 to 2 minutes until cheese has melted.

6. Serve.

Nutrition :

355 Calories; 28 g Fats; 18.6 g Protein; 5.7 g Net Carb; 2.3 g Fiber;

Egg McMuffin Sandwich with Avocado and Bacon

Preparation Time : 10 minutes;

Cooking Time : 15 minutes;

Servings : 2

Ingredients

- 2 eggs, yolks and egg whites separated
- 1/3 cup grated parmesan cheese
- 2 oz cream cheese, softened
- 2 slices of bacon
- ½ of avocado, sliced
- Seasoning:
- 2/3 tsp salt
- 1 tsp avocado oil

Directions:

1. Take a medium bowl, place egg yolks in it, add cream cheese, parmesan, and salt and whisk by using an electric blender until smooth.

2. Take another medium bowl, add egg whites, beat until stiff peaks form and then fold egg whites into egg yolk mixture until combined.

3. Take a skillet pan, place it over medium heat, add oil and when hot, add one-fourth of the batter, spread it into a 1-inch thick pancake, and then fry got 2 minutes per side until golden brown.

4. When done, let sandwiches cool for 5 minutes, top two muffins with bacon and avocado slices, cover the top with another muffin, and then serve as desired.

Nutrition :

355 Calories; 28 g Fats; 18.6 g Protein; 5.7 g Net Carb; 2.3 g Fiber;

Cheese & Spinach Stuffed Chicken

PREPARATION TIME : 50 MINUTES

COOKING TIME : 40 MINUTES

SERVINGS: 4

Ingredients

- 4 chicken breasts, boneless and skinless
- ½ cup mozzarella cheese
- 1 ½ cups Parmesan cheese, shredded
- 6 ounces cream cheese
- 2 cups spinach, chopped
- A pinch of nutmeg
- ½ tsp garlic, minced
- **<u>Breading</u>**
- 2 eggs, beaten
- 1/3 cup almond flour
- 2 tbsp. olive oil
- ½ tsp parsley
- 1/3 cup Parmesan cheese
- A pinch of onion powder

Directions

1. Pound the chicken until it doubles in size. Mix cream cheese, spinach, mozzarella cheese, nutmeg, and salt, pepper, and Parmesan cheese in a bowl. Divide the mixture between the chicken breasts and spread it out evenly. Wrap the chicken in a plastic wrap. Refrigerate for 15 minutes.

2. Preheat the oven to 370 F.

3. Beat the eggs and set aside. Combine all of the other breading ingredients in a bowl. Dip the chicken in eggs first, then in the breading mixture.

4. Warm the olive oil in a pan over medium heat. Cook the chicken in the pan until browned, about 5-6 minutes. Place on a lined baking sheet, and bake for 20 minutes. Serve.

Nutrition

Calories 491, Net Carbs 3.5g, Fat 36g, Protein 38g

Asian Chicken with Fresh Lime-Peanut Sauce

PREPARATION TIME : 1 HOUR AND 30 MINUTES

COOKING TIME : 40 MINUTES

SERVINGS: 6

Ingredients

- 1 tbsp. wheat-free soy sauce
- 1 tbsp. sugar-free fish sauce
- 1 tbsp. lime juice
- 1 tsp coriander
- 1 tsp garlic, minced
- 1 tsp ginger, minced
- 1 tbsp. olive oil
- 1 tbsp. rice wine vinegar
- 1 tsp cayenne pepper
- 1 tbsp. erythritol
- 6 chicken thighs
- **Sauce:**
- ½ cup peanut butter
- 1 tsp garlic, minced
- 1 tbsp. lime juice

- 2 tbsp. water
- 1 tsp ginger, minced
- 1 tbsp. jalapeño, chopped
- 2 tbsp. rice wine vinegar
- 2 tbsp. erythritol
- 1 tbsp. fish sauce

Directions

1. Combine all of the chicken ingredients in a large Ziploc bag.
2. Seal the bag and shake to combine.
3. Refrigerate for about 1 hour.
4. Remove from the fridge about 15 minutes before cooking.
5. Preheat the grill to medium, and grill the chicken for about 7 minutes per side.
6. Meanwhile, whisk together all of the sauce ingredients in a mixing bowl.
7. Serve the chicken drizzled with peanut sauce.

Nutrition

Calories 492, Net Carbs 3g, Fat 36g, Protein 35g

Bacon-Wrapped Chicken with Grilled Asparagus

PREPARATION TIME : 50 MINUTES

COOKING TIME : 40 MINUTES

SERVINGS: 4

Ingredients

- 2 tbsp. fresh lemon juice
- 6 chicken breasts
- 8 bacon slices
- 1 tbsp. olive oil
- 1 lb. asparagus spears
- 3 tbsp. olive oil
- Salt and black pepper to taste
- Manchego cheese for topping

Directions

1. Preheat the oven to 400 F.
2. Season chicken breasts with salt and black pepper, and wrap 2 bacon slices around each chicken breast. Arrange on a baking sheet that is lined with

parchment paper, drizzle with oil, and bake for 25-30 minutes until bacon is brown and crispy.

3. Preheat the grill.
4. Brush the asparagus spears with olive oil and season with salt. Grill turning frequently until slightly charred, 5-10 minutes.
5. Remove to a plate and drizzle with lemon juice. Grate over Manchego cheese so that it melts a little on contact with the hot asparagus and forms a cheesy dressing.

Nutrition

Calories 468, Net Carbs 2g, Fat 38g, Protein 26g

Spicy Cheese Chicken Soup

PREPARATION TIME : 15 MINUTES

COOKING TIME : 40 MINUTES

SERVINGS: 4

Ingredients

- ½ cup salsa enchilada verde
- 2 cups chicken, cooked and shredded
- 2 cups chicken or bone broth
- 1 cup cheddar cheese, shredded
- 4 ounces cream cheese
- ½ tsp chili powder
- ½ tsp cumin, ground
- ½ tsp fresh cilantro, chopped
- Salt and black pepper to taste

Directions

1. Combine the cream cheese, salsa verde, and broth in a food processor.
2. Pulse until smooth. Transfer the mixture to a pot and place over medium heat.
3. Cook until hot, but do not bring to a boil.

4. Add chicken, chili powder, and cumin, and cook for about 3-5 minutes, or until it is heated through. Stir in Cheddar cheese. Season with salt and pepper to taste.

5. Serve hot in individual bowls sprinkled with fresh cilantro.

Nutrition

Calories 346, Net Carbs 3g, Fat 23g, Protein 25g

Bok Choy Caesar Salad with Chicken

PREPARATION TIME : 1 HOUR AND 20 MINUTES

COOKING TIME : 40 MINUTES

SERVINGS: 4

Ingredients

- **<u>Chicken</u>**
- 4 chicken thighs, boneless and skinless
- ¼ cup lemon juice
- 2 garlic cloves, minced
- 2 tbsp. olive oil
- **<u>Salad</u>**
- ½ cup caesar salad dressing, sugar-free
- 2 tbsp. olive oil
- 12 bok choy leaves
- 3 Parmesan cheese crisps
- Parmesan cheese, grated or garnishing

Directions

1. Combine the chicken ingredients in a Ziploc bag. Seal the bag, shake to combine, and refrigerate for 1 hour.
2. Preheat the grill to medium heat, and grill the chicken about 4 minutes per side.
3. Cut bok choy leaves lengthwise, and brush it with oil. Grill for about 3 minutes. Place on a serving platter. Top with the chicken, and drizzle the dressing over. Sprinkle with Parmesan cheese and finish with Parmesan crisps to serve.

Nutrition

Calories 529, Net Carbs 5g, Fat 39g, Protein 33g

Chicken & Spinach Gratin

PREPARATION TIME : 45 MINUTES

COOKING TIME : 40 MINUTES

SERVINGS: 6

Ingredients

- 6 chicken breasts, skinless and boneless
- 1 tsp mixed spice seasoning
- Pink salt and black pepper to season
- 2 loose cups baby spinach
- 3 tsp olive oil
- 4 oz cream cheese, cubed
- 1 ¼ cups mozzarella cheese, shredded
- 4 tbsp. water

Directions

1. Preheat oven to 375 F.
2. Season chicken with spice mix, salt, and black pepper. Pat with your hands to have the seasoning stick on the chicken.
3. Put in the casserole dish and layer spinach over the chicken.

4. Mix the oil with cream cheese, mozzarella, salt, and black pepper and stir in water a tablespoon at a time.

5. Pour the mixture over the chicken and cover the pot with aluminum foil.

6. Bake for 20 minutes, remove foil and continue cooking for 15 minutes until a beautiful golden brown color is formed on top.

7. Take out and allow sitting for 5 minutes. Serve warm with braised asparagus.

Nutrition

Calories 340, Net Carbs 1g, Fat 30.2g, Protein 15g

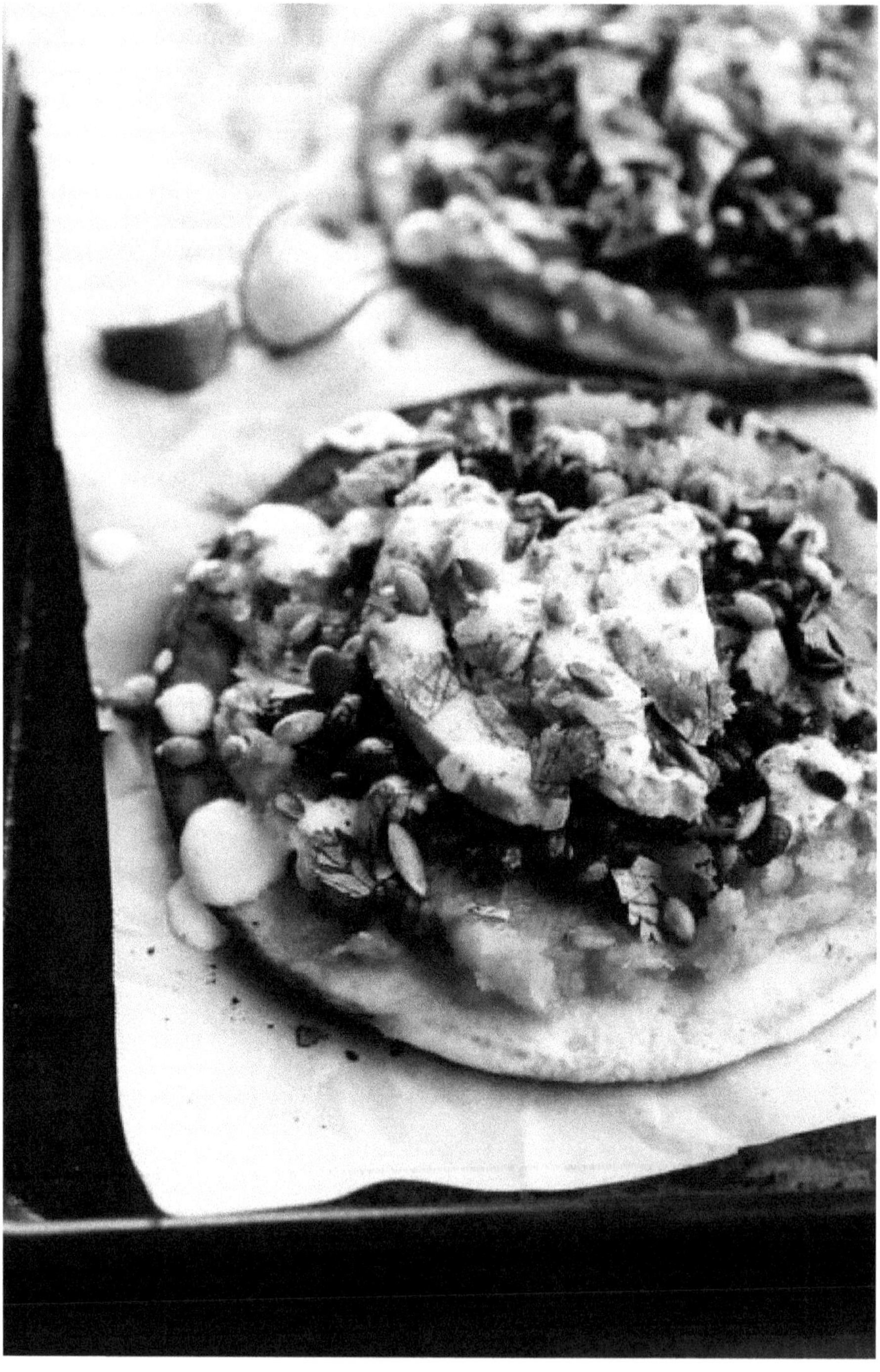

Chili Chicken Kabobs with Tahini Dressing

PREPARATION TIME : 20 MINUTES+ 2 HOURS REFRIGERATION

COOKING TIME : 10 MINUTES

SERVINGS: 6

Ingredients

- 3 tbsp. soy sauce
- 1 tbsp. ginger-garlic paste
- 2 tbsp. swerve brown sugar
- 2 tbsp. olive oil
- 3 chicken breasts, cut into bite-sized cubes
- ½ cup tahini
- ½ tsp garlic powder
- Salt and chili pepper to taste

Directions

1. In a bowl, whisk soy sauce, ginger-garlic paste, swerve brown sugar, chili pepper, and olive oil. Put the chicken in a zipper bag, pour the marinade over,

seal, and shake for an even coat. Marinate in the fridge for 2 hours.

2. Preheat a grill to 400 F and thread the chicken on skewers. Cook for 10 minutes in total with three to four turnings to be golden brown. Plate them.

3. Mix the tahini, garlic powder, salt, and ¼ cup of warm water in a bowl. Serve the chicken skewers and tahini dressing with cauliflower fried rice.

Nutrition

Calories 225, Net Carbs 2g, Fat 17.4g, Protein 15g

Chicken with Eggplant & Tomatoes

PREPARATION TIME : 25 MINUTES

COOKING TIME : 10 MINUTES

SERVINGS: 4

Ingredients

- 2 tbsp. ghee
- 1 lb. chicken thighs
- Salt and black pepper to taste
- 2 cloves garlic, minced
- 1 (14 oz) can whole tomatoes
- 1 eggplant, diced
- 10 fresh basil leaves, chopped + extra to garnish

Directions

1. Melt ghee in a saucepan over medium heat, season the chicken with salt and black pepper, and fry for 4 minutes on each side until golden brown. Remove the chicken onto a plate.

2. Sauté the garlic in the ghee for 2 minutes, pour in the tomatoes, and cook covered for 8 minutes. Include the eggplant and basil. Cook for 4 minutes.
3. Season the sauce with salt and black pepper, stir and add the chicken. Coat with sauce and simmer for 3 minutes.
4. Serve chicken with sauce on a bed of squash pasta garnished with basil.

Nutrition

Calories 468, Net Carbs 2g, Fat 39.5g, Protein 26g

Tasty Chicken with Brussel Sprouts

PREPARATION TIME : 120 MINUTES

COOKING TIME : 40 MINUTES

SERVINGS: 8

Ingredients

- 5 pounds whole chicken
- 1 bunch oregano
- 1 bunch thyme
- 1 tbsp. marjoram
- 1 tbsp. parsley
- 1 tbsp. olive oil
- 2 pounds Brussel sprouts
- 1 lemon
- 4 tbsp. butter

Directions

1. Preheat your oven to 450 F.
2. Stuff the chicken with oregano, thyme, and lemon.
3. Make sure the wings are tucked over and behind.

4. Roast for 15 minutes. Reduce the heat to 325 F, and cook for 40 minutes.
5. Spread the butter over the chicken and sprinkle parsley and marjoram.
6. Add the Brussel sprouts. Return to oven and bake for 40 more minutes.
7. Let sit for 10 minutes before carving.

Nutrition

Calories 430, Net Carbs 5g, Fat 32g, Protein 30g

Weekend Chicken with Grapefruit & Lemon

PREPARATION TIME : 30 MINUTES

COOKING TIME : 40 MINUTES

SERVINGS: 4

Ingredients

- 1 cup omission IPA
- A pinch of garlic powder
- 1 tsp grapefruit zest
- 3 tbsp. lemon juice
- ½ tsp coriander, ground
- 1 tbsp. fish sauce
- 2 tbsp. butter
- ¼ tsp xanthan gum
- 3 tbsp. swerve sweetener
- 20 chicken wing pieces
- Salt and black pepper to taste

Directions

1. Combine lemon juice and zest, fish sauce, coriander, omission IPA, sweetener, and garlic powder in a saucepan.
2. Bring to a boil, cover, lower the heat, and let simmer for 10 minutes.
3. Stir in the butter and xanthan gum. Set aside. Season the wings with some salt and pepper.
4. Preheat the grill and cook for 5 minutes per side.
5. Serve topped with the sauce.

Nutrition

Calories 365, Net Carbs 4g, Fat 25g, Protein 21g

Rosemary Chicken with Avocado Sauce

PREPARATION TIME : 22 MINUTES

COOKING TIME : 30 MINUTES

SERVINGS: 4

Ingredients

- 1 avocado pitted
- ½ cup mayonnaise
- 3 tbsp. ghee
- 4 chicken breasts
- Salt and black pepper to taste
- 1 cup rosemary, chopped
- ½ cup chicken broth

Directions

1. Spoon avocado, mayonnaise, and salt into a food processor and puree until a smooth sauce is derived. Adjust the taste with salt. Pour sauce into a jar and refrigerate.

2. Melt ghee in a large skillet, season chicken with salt and black pepper, and fry for 4 minutes on each side to a golden brown. Remove chicken to a plate.
3. Pour the broth in the same skillet and add the cilantro. Bring to simmer covered for 3 minutes and add the chicken. Cover, and cook on low heat for 5 minutes until the liquid has reduced and chicken is fragrant.
4. Dish chicken only into serving plates and spoon the mayo-avocado sauce over.
5. Serve warm with buttered green beans and baby carrots.

Nutrition

Calories 398, Net Carbs 4g, Fat 32g, Protein 24g

Turkey Patties with Cucumber Salsa

PREPARATION TIME : 30 MINUTES

COOKING TIME : 40 MINUTES

SERVINGS: 4

Ingredients

- 2 spring onions, thinly sliced
- 1 pound turkey, ground
- 1 egg
- 2 garlic cloves, minced
- 1 tbsp. herbs, chopped
- 1 small chili pepper, deseeded and diced
- 2 tbsp. ghee
- **Cucumber Salsa:**
- 1 tbsp. apple cider vinegar
- 1 tbsp. dill, chopped
- 1 garlic clove, minced
- 2 cucumbers, grated
- 1 cup sour cream
- 1 jalapeño pepper, minced
- 2 tbsp. olive oil

Directions

1. Place all of the turkey ingredients, except the ghee, in a bowl. Mix to combine. Make patties out of the mixture.

2. Melt ghee in a skillet over medium heat. Cook the patties for 3 minutes per side.

3. Place all of the salsa ingredients in a bowl and mix to combine. Serve the patties topped with salsa.

Nutrition

Calories 475, Net Carbs 5g, Fat 38g, Protein 26g

Pancakes

Preparation Time : 5 minutes

Cooking Time : 6 minutes

Servings : 2

Ingredients

- ¼ cup almond flour
- 1 ½ tbsp. unsalted butter
- 2 oz cream cheese, softened
- 2 eggs

Directions:

1. Take a bowl, crack eggs in it, whisk well until fluffy, and then whisk in flour and cream cheese until well combined.
2. Take a skillet pan, place it over medium heat, add butter and when it melts, drop pancake batter in four sections, spread it evenly, and cook for 2 minutes per side until brown.
3. Serve.

Nutrition :

166.8 Calories; 15 g Fats; 5.8 g Protein; 1.8 g Net Carb; 0.8 g Fiber;

Cheese Roll-Ups

Preparation Time : 5 minutes

Cooking Time : 0 minutes;

Servings : 2

Ingredients

- 2 oz mozzarella cheese, sliced, full-fat
- 1-ounce butter, unsalted

Directions:

1. Cut cheese into slices and then cut butter into thin slices.
2. Top each cheese slice with a slice of butter, roll it and then serve.

Nutrition :

166 Calories; 15 g Fats; 6.5 g Protein; 2 g Net Carb; 0 g Fiber;

Scrambled Eggs with Spinach and Cheese

Preparation Time : 5 minutes

Cooking Time : 5 minutes;

Servings : 2

Ingredients

- 2 oz spinach
- 2 eggs
- 1 tbsp. coconut oil
- 2 tbsp. grated mozzarella cheese, full-fat
- Seasoning:
- ¼ tsp salt
- 1/8 tsp ground black pepper
- 1/8 tsp red pepper flakes

Directions:

1. Take a medium bowl, crack eggs in it, add salt and black pepper and whisk until combined.
2. Take a medium skillet pan, place it over medium heat, add oil and when hot, add spinach and cook for 1 minute until leaves wilt.

3. Pour eggs over spinach, stir and cook for 1 minute until just set.

4. Stir in cheese, then remove the pan from heat and sprinkle red pepper flakes on top.

5. Serve.

Nutrition :

171 Calories; 14 g Fats; 9.2 g Protein; 1.1 g Net Carb; 1.7 g Fiber;

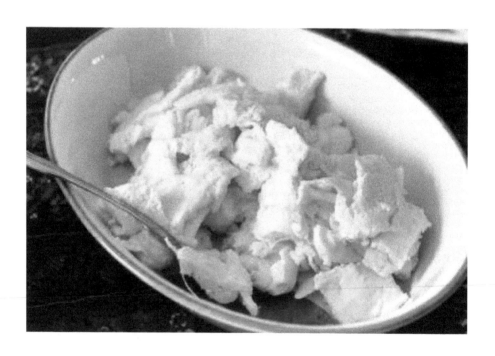

Egg Wraps

Preparation Time : 5 minutes

Cooking Time : 5 minutes;

Servings : 2

Ingredients

- 2 eggs
- 1 tbsp. coconut oil
- Seasoning:
- ¼ tsp salt
- 1/8 tsp ground black pepper

Directions:

Take a medium bowl, crack eggs in it, add salt and black pepper, and then whisk until blended.

Take a frying pan, place it over medium-low heat, add coconut oil and when it melts, pour in half of the egg, spread it evenly into a thin layer by rotating the pan and cook for 2 minutes.

Then flip the pan, cook for 1 minute, and transfer to a plate.

Repeat with the remaining egg to make another wrap, then roll each egg wrap and serve.

Nutrition :

68 Calories; 4.7 g Fats; 5.5 g Protein; 0.5 g Net Carb; 0 g Fiber;

Chaffles with Poached Eggs

Preparation Time : 5 minutes

Cooking Time : 10 minutes;

Servings : 2

Ingredients

- 2 tsp coconut flour
- ½ cup shredded cheddar cheese, full-fat
- 3 eggs
- Seasoning:
- ¼ tsp salt
- 1/8 tsp ground black pepper

Directions:

1. Switch on a mini waffle maker and let it preheat for 5 minutes.
2. Meanwhile, take a medium bowl, place all the ingredients in it, reserving 2 eggs and then mix by using an immersion blender until smooth.
3. Ladle the batter evenly into the waffle maker, shut with lid, and let it cook for 3 to 4 minutes until firm and golden brown.

4. Meanwhile, prepare poached eggs, and for this, take a medium bowl half full with water, place it over medium heat and bring it to a boil.

5. Then crack an egg in a ramekin, carefully pour it into the boiling water and cook for 3 minutes.

6. Transfer egg to a plate lined with paper towels by using a slotted spoon and repeat with the other egg.

7. Top chaffles with poached eggs, season with salt and black pepper, and then serve.

Nutrition :

265 Calories; 18.5 g Fats; 17.6 g Protein; 3.4 g Net Carb; 6 g Fiber;

Chaffle with Scrambled Eggs

Preparation Time : 5 minutes

Cooking Time : 10 minutes;

Servings: 2

Ingredients

- 2 tsp coconut flour
- ½ cup shredded cheddar cheese, full-fat
- 3 eggs
- 1-ounce butter, unsalted
- Seasoning:
- ¼ tsp salt
- 1/8 tsp ground black pepper
- 1/8 tsp dried oregano

Directions:

1. Switch on a mini waffle maker and let it preheat for 5 minutes.
2. Meanwhile, take a medium bowl, place all the ingredients in it, reserving 2 eggs and then mix by using an immersion blender until smooth.

3. Ladle the batter evenly into the waffle maker, shut with lid, and let it cook for 3 to 4 minutes until firm and golden brown.
4. Meanwhile, prepare scrambled eggs and for this, take a medium bowl, crack the eggs in it and whisk them with a fork until frothy, and then season with salt and black pepper.
5. Take a medium skillet pan, place it over medium heat, add butter and when it melts, pour in eggs and cook for 2 minutes until creamy, stirring continuously.
6. Top chaffles with scrambled eggs, sprinkle with oregano, and then serve.

Nutrition :

265 Calories; 18.5 g Fats; 17.6 g Protein; 3.4 g Net Carb; 6 g Fiber;

Sheet Pan Eggs with Mushrooms and Spinach

Preparation Time : 5 minutes

Cooking Time : 12 minutes;

Servings : 2

Ingredients

- 2 eggs
- 1 tsp chopped jalapeno pepper
- 1 tbsp. chopped mushrooms
- 1 tbsp. chopped spinach
- 1 tbsp. chopped chard
- Seasoning:
- 1/3 tsp salt
- 1/4 tsp ground black pepper

Directions:

1. Turn on the oven, then set it to 350 degrees F and let it preheat.
2. Take a medium bowl, crack eggs in it, add salt and black pepper, then add all the vegetables and stir until combined.

3. Take a medium sheet ball or rimmed baking sheet, grease it with oil, pour prepared egg batter on it, and then bake for 10 to 12 minutes until done.

4. Cut egg into two squares and then serve.

Nutrition :

165 Calories; 10.7 g Fats; 14 g Protein; 1.5 g Net Carb; 0.5 g Fiber;

No Bread Breakfast Sandwich

Preparation Time : 10 minutes

Cooking Time : 15 minutes;

Servings : 2

Ingredients

- 2 slices of ham
- 4 eggs
- 1 tsp tabasco sauce
- 3 tbsp. butter, unsalted
- 2 tsp grated mozzarella cheese
- Seasoning:
- ¼ tsp salt
- 1/8 tsp ground black pepper

Directions:

1. Take a frying pan, place it over medium heat, add butter and when it melt, crack an egg in it and fry for 2 to 3 minutes until cooked to desired level.
2. Transfer fried egg to a plate, fry remaining eggs in the same manner and when done, season eggs with salt and black pepper.

3. Prepare the sandwich and for this, use a fried egg as a base for sandwich, then top with a ham slice, sprinkle with a tsp of ham and cover with another fried egg.
4. Place egg into the pan, return it over low heat and let it cook until cheese melts.
5. Prepare another sandwich in the same manner and then serve.

Nutrition :

180 Calories; 15 g Fats; 10 g Protein; 1 g Net Carb; 0 g Fiber;

Scrambled Eggs with Basil and Butter

Preparation Time : 5 minutes

Cooking Time : 5 minutes;

Servings : 2

Ingredients

- 1 tbsp. chopped basil leaves
- 2 tbsp. butter, unsalted
- 2 tbsp. grated cheddar cheese
- 2 eggs
- 2 tbsp. whipping cream
- Seasoning:
- 1/8 tsp salt
- 1/8 tsp ground black pepper

Directions:

1. Take a medium bowl, crack eggs in it, add salt, black pepper, cheese and cream and whisk until combined.
2. Take a medium pan, place it over low heat, add butter and when it melts, pour in the egg mixture and cook

for 2 to 3 minutes until eggs have scrambled to the desired level.

3. When done, distribute scrambled eggs between two plates, top with basil leaves and then serve.

Nutrition :

320 Calories; 29 g Fats; 13 g Protein; 1.5 g Net Carb; 0 g Fiber;

Bacon, and Eggs

Preparation Time : 5 minutes

Cooking Time : 10 minutes;

Servings : 2

Ingredients

- 2 eggs
- 4 slices of turkey bacon
- ¼ tsp salt
- ¼ tsp ground black pepper

Directions:

1. Take a skillet pan, place it over medium heat, add bacon slices in it and cook for 5 minutes until crispy.
2. Transfer bacon slices to a plate and set aside until required, reserving the fat in the pan.
3. Cook the egg in the pan one at a time, and for this, crack an egg in the pan and cook for 2 to 3 minutes or more until the egg has cooked to desire level.
4. Transfer egg to a plate and cook the other egg in the same manner.
5. Season eggs with salt and black pepper and then serve with cooked bacon.

Nutrition :

136 Calories; 11 g Fats; 7.5 g Protein; 1 g Net Carb; 0 g Fiber

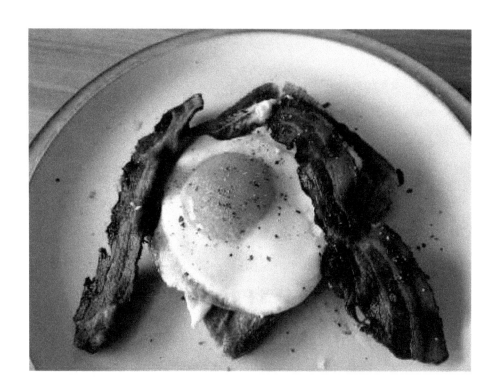

Boiled Eggs

Preparation Time : 5 minutes

Cooking Time : 10 minutes;

Servings : 2

Ingredients

- 2 eggs
- ½ of a medium avocado
- Seasoning:
- ¼ tsp salt
- ¼ tsp ground black pepper

Directions:

1. Place a medium pot over medium heat, fill it half full with water and bring it to boil.
2. Then carefully place the eggs in the boiling water and boil the eggs for 5 minutes until soft-boiled, 8 minutes for medium-boiled, and 10 minutes for hard-boiled.
3. When eggs have boiled, transfer them to a bowl containing chilled water and let them rest for 5 minutes.
4. Then crack the eggs with a spoon and peel them.

5. Cut each egg into slices, season with salt and black pepper, and serve with diced avocado.

Nutrition :

112 Calories; 9.5 g Fats; 5.5 g Protein; 1 g Net Carb; 0 g Fiber;

Beef with Cabbage Noodles

Preparation Time : 5 minutes

Cooking Time : 18 minutes

Servings : 2

Ingredients

- 4 oz ground beef
- 1 cup chopped cabbage
- 4 oz tomato sauce
- ½ tsp minced garlic
- ½ cup of water
- Seasoning:
- ½ tbsp. coconut oil
- ½ tsp salt
- ¼ tsp Italian seasoning
- 1/8 tsp dried basil

Directions:

1. Take a skillet pan, place it over medium heat, add oil and when hot, add beef and cook for 5 minutes until nicely browned.

2. Meanwhile, prepare the cabbage and for it, slice the cabbage into thin shred.

3. When the beef has cooked, add garlic, season with salt, basil, and Italian seasoning, stir well and continue cooking for 3 minutes until beef has thoroughly cooked.

4. Pour in tomato sauce and water, stir well and bring the mixture to boil.

5. Then reduce heat to medium-low level, add cabbage, stir well until well mixed and simmer for 3 to 5 minutes until cabbage is softened, covering the pan.

6. Uncover the pan and continue simmering the beef until most of the cooking liquid has evaporated.

7. Serve.

Nutrition :

188.5 Calories; 12.5 g Fats; 15.5 g Protein; 2.5 g Net Carb; 1 g Fiber;

Roast Beef and Mozzarella Plate

Preparation Time : 5 minutes

Cooking Time : 0 minutes;

Servings : 2

Ingredients

- 4 slices of roast beef
- ½ ounce chopped lettuce
- 1 avocado, pitted
- 2 oz mozzarella cheese, cubed
- ½ cup mayonnaise
- Seasoning:
- ¼ tsp salt
- 1/8 tsp ground black pepper
- 2 tbsp. avocado oil

Directions:

1. Scoop out flesh from avocado and divide it evenly between two plates.
2. Add slices of roast beef, lettuce, and cheese and then sprinkle with salt and black pepper.
3. Serve with avocado oil and mayonnaise.

Nutrition :

267.7 Calories; 24.5 g Fats; 9.5 g Protein; 1.5 g Net Carb; 2 g
Fiber;

Beef and Broccoli

Preparation Time : 5 minutes

Cooking Time : 10 minutes;

Servings : 2

Ingredients

- 6 slices of beef roast, cut into strips
- 1 scallion, chopped
- 3 oz broccoli florets, chopped
- 1 tbsp. avocado oil
- 1 tbsp. butter, unsalted
- Seasoning:
- ¼ tsp salt
- 1/8 tsp ground black pepper
- 1 ½ tbsp. soy sauce
- 3 tbsp. chicken broth

Directions:

1. Take a medium skillet pan, place it over medium heat, add oil and when hot, add beef strips and cook for 2 minutes until hot.
2. Transfer beef to a plate, add scallion to the pan, then add butter and cook for 3 minutes until tender.

3. Add remaining ingredients, stir until mixed, switch heat to the low level and simmer for 3 to 4 minutes until broccoli is tender.

4. Return beef to the pan, stir until well combined and cook for 1 minute.

5. Serve.

Nutrition :

245 Calories; 15.7 g Fats; 21.6 g Protein; 1.7 g Net Carb; 1.3 g Fiber;

Garlic Herb Beef Roast

Preparation Time : 5 minutes

Cooking Time : 10 minutes;

Servings : 2

Ingredients

- 6 slices of beef roast
- ½ tsp garlic powder
- 1/3 tsp dried thyme
- ¼ tsp dried rosemary
- 2 tbsp. butter, unsalted
- Seasoning:
- 1/3 tsp salt
- 1/4 tsp ground black pepper

Directions:

1. Prepare the spice mix and for this, take a small bowl, place garlic powder, thyme, rosemary, salt, and black pepper and then stir until mixed.
2. Sprinkle spice mix on the beef roast.
3. Take a medium skillet pan, place it over medium heat, add butter and when it melts, add beef roast

and then cook for 5 to 8 minutes until golden brown and cooked.

4. Serve.

Nutrition :

140 Calories; 12.7 g Fats; 5.5 g Protein; 0.1 g Net Carb; 0.2 g Fiber;

Sprouts Stir-fry with Kale, Broccoli, and Beef

Preparation Time : 5 minutes

Cooking Time : 8 minutes;

Servings : 2

Ingredients

- 3 slices of beef roast, chopped
- 2 oz Brussels sprouts, halved
- 4 oz broccoli florets
- 3 oz kale
- 1 ½ tbsp. butter, unsalted
- 1/8 tsp red pepper flakes
- Seasoning:
- ¼ tsp garlic powder
- ¼ tsp salt
- 1/8 tsp ground black pepper

Directions:

1. Take a medium skillet pan, place it over medium heat, add ¾ tbsp. butter and when it melts, add

broccoli florets and sprouts, sprinkle with garlic powder, and cook for 2 minutes.

2. Season vegetables with salt and red pepper flakes, add chopped beef, stir until mixed and continue cooking for 3 minutes until browned on one side.

3. Then add kale along with remaining butter, flip the vegetables and cook for 2 minutes until kale leaves wilts.

4. Serve.

Nutrition :

125 Calories; 9.4 g Fats; 4.8 g Protein; 1.7 g Net Carb; 2.6 g Fiber;

Beef and Vegetable Skillet

Preparation Time : 5 minutes

Cooking Time : 15 minutes

Servings : 2

Ingredients

- 3 oz spinach, chopped
- ½ pound ground beef
- 2 slices of bacon, diced
- 2 oz chopped asparagus
- Seasoning:
- 3 tbsp. coconut oil
- 2 tsp dried thyme
- 2/3 tsp salt
- ½ tsp ground black pepper

Directions:

1. Take a skillet pan, place it over medium heat, add oil and when hot, add beef and bacon and cook for 5 to 7 minutes until slightly browned.
2. Then add asparagus and spinach, sprinkle with thyme, stir well and cook for 7 to 10 minutes until thoroughly cooked.

3. Season skillet with salt and black pepper and serve.

Nutrition :

332.5 Calories; 26 g Fats; 23.5 g Protein; 1.5 g Net Carb; 1 g Fiber;

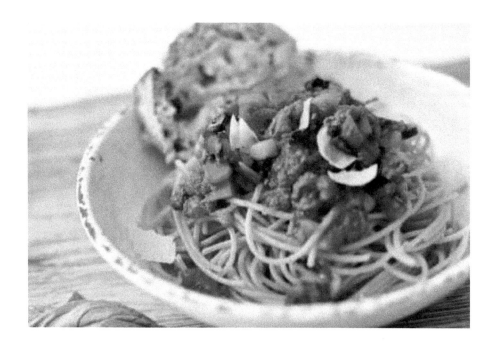

30-Day Meal Plan

Days	Breakfast	Lunch	Dinner	Snacks
1	Bacon Cheeseburger Waffles	Buttered Cod	Baked Crispy Chicken	Fluffy Bites
2	Keto Breakfast Cheesecake	Salmon with Red Curry Sauce	Italian Chicken	Coconut Fudge
3	Egg-Crust Pizza	Salmon Teriyaki	Chicken & Carrots	Nutmeg Nougat
4	Breakfast Roll Ups	Pesto Shrimp with Zucchini Noodles	Lemon & Herb Chicken	Sweet Almond Bites
5	Basic Opie Rolls	Crab Cakes	Chicken & Avocado Salad	Strawberry Cheesecake Minis
6	Cream Cheese Pancake	Tuna Salad	Chicken Bowl	Cocoa Brownies
7	Blueberry Coconut Porridge	Keto Frosty	Chicken with Bacon & Ranch Sauce	Chocolate Orange Bites
8	Cauliflower Hash Browns	Keto Shake	Creamy Chicken & Mushroo	Caramel Cones

			m	
9	**Keto Rolls**	Keto Fat Bombs	Mozzarell a Chicken	Cinnamon Bites
10	**Breakfast Roll Ups**	Avocado Ice Pops	Chicken Parmesan	Sweet Chai Bites
11	**Almond Flour Pancakes**	Carrot Balls	Pasta	Easy Vanilla Bombs
12	**Avocado Toast**	Coconut Crack Bars	Crab Melt	Marinated Eggs.
13	**Chicken Avocado Egg Bacon Salad**	Strawberry Ice Cream	Spinach Frittata	Sausage and Cheese Dip.
14	**Bacon Wrapped Chicken Breast**	Key Lime Pudding	Halloumi Time	Tasty Onion and Cauliflowe r Dip.
15	**Egg Salad**	Easy Meatballs	Hash Browns	Pesto Crackers.
16	**Blueberry Muffins**	Chicken in Sweet and Sour Sauce with Corn Salad	Poblano Peppers	Pumpkin Muffins.
17	**Bacon Hash**	Chinese Chicken Salad	Mushroo m Omelet	Cheesy Salami Snack
18	**Bagels With Cheese**	Chicken Salad	Tuna Casserole	Creamy Mango and Mint Dip
19	**Cauli Flitters**	Tofu Meat and Salad	Goat Cheese	Hot Red Chili and

			Frittata	Garlic Chutney
20	**Scrambled Eggs**	Asparagus and Pistachios Vinaigrette	Pasta	Red Chilies and Onion Chutney
21	**Frittata with Spinach**	Turkey Meatballs	Muffins	Fast Guacamole
22	**Cheese Omelet**	Easy Meatballs	Meaty Salad	Coconut Dill Dip
23	**Capicola Egg Cups**	Chicken, Bacon and Avocado Cloud Sandwiches	Pasta	Creamy Crab Dip
24	**Breakfast Roll Ups**	Roasted Lemon Chicken Sandwich	Crab Soup	Creamy Cheddar and Bacon Spread with Almonds
25	**Overnight "noats"**	Keto-Friendly Skillet Pepperoni Pizza	Southern Bean Casserole	Green Tabasco Devilled Eggs
26	**Frozen keto coffee**	Cheesy Chicken Cauliflower	Low-Carb Okra	Herbed Cheese Balls
27	**Easy Skillet Pancakes**	Chicken Soup	Cauli Rice	Cheesy Salami Snack
28	**Quick Keto**	Chicken	Southern	Pesto &

		Avocado Salad	Fried Chicken	Olive Fat Bombs
	Blender Muffins			
29	**Keto Everything Bagels**	Chicken Broccoli Dinner	Low-Carb Lasagna	Cheesy Broccoli Nuggets
30	**Turmeric Chicken and Kale Salad with Food, Lemon and Honey**	Easy Meatballs	Low-Carb Spaghetti Bolognese	Salmon Fat Bombs

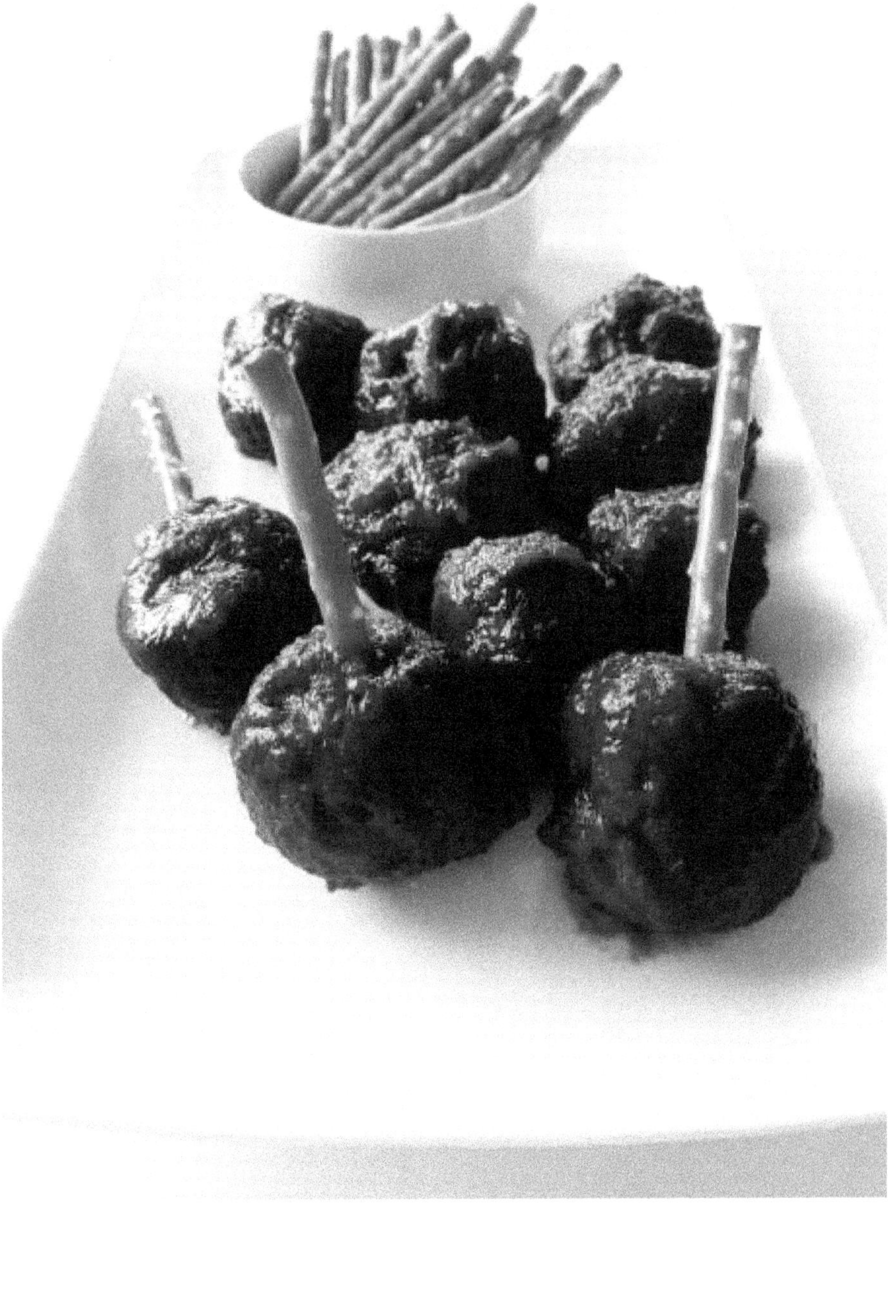

Lightning Source UK Ltd.
Milton Keynes UK
UKHW021018240621
386074UK00004B/200